SELLING YOUR DENTAL PRACTICE:
preparation, processes and procedures to maximize the value of your business to buyers

Table of Contents

Foreword

My name is Dr. Kevin Coughlin, and I'm a general dentist who owns 14 practices in Western Massachusetts, employing 150 people.

I've practiced the art and science of dentistry and business for over 3 decades.

The focus of this mini-book is to help dentists prepare their greatest asset - their practice - for sale.

This is the third in a series of books written for dentists at every stage of their careers. In the first book of this series, I discussed how a recent graduate starts their practice, gets their first job, and navigates the ups and downs of that initial transition.

The second book showed dentists how to grow their practices based on the SPECIAL formula.

- Scheduling
- Production
- Employees
- Collection
- Internal controls
- Associates
- Liability

I discussed how dentists can make their practices special; how they can grow their practices exponentially, and outlined the processes and procedures to improve their financial situation.

In this final installment, I'm going to focus on the practitioner who, in most cases, is in their late 50s or early 60s, and is considering selling their dental practice.

Let's start with an analogy we can all easily understand. You would never begin a clinical case without first having a comprehensive knowledge of a patient's past medical and dental history, as well as their chief complaint and all the radiographs, diagnostic photos, diagnostic impressions, periodontal charting, a risk assessment, financial arrangements, etc.

In essence, you gather as much information as you can before you do anything. Take that same approach to the sale of your practice and you will likely save yourself headaches and also see a better ROI when the paperwork is all signed, sealed and delivered.

To get that maximum return, you need preparation. This process should start the day you graduate from dental school because the value of your practice is tied to the processes and procedures you put in place throughout your career.

When a potential purchaser is evaluating your practice, they are not simply paying for a patient list. They are looking at your overall business model. So, how you run your business at every level affects the perceived value to these potential buyers.

The procedures associated with planning your dental practice should always have a strategy that includes the eventual sale of that asset. For most of us, our dental practice will be the largest asset. In order to get the best value involving the least amount of stress, it's critical that you fully understand the four stages of a dental practice.

Four stages of a dental practice

- **Stage 1**. This stage is generally going to be a de novo option. You either start off from scratch with your own practice, or buy in/out an existing practice.
- **Stage 2**. This is the growth stage of your practice. Patients will opt for or against your practice based on your style and type of practice you have created.
- **Stage 3.** Stage three is when your practice reaches maturity. It has reached its intended goals and objectives.
- **Stage 4.** This is the redevelopment stage, which means you either let the practice die naturally or you take steps to maximize its value and prepare it for sale. The reason for maximizing the value would be so you can get the best return on your investment.

As you are reading this book, I'm going to assume that you have decided to maximize the value of your practice to get the best return on your investment.

During my long career, I've grown my business to include 14 practices - which were then sold for a tidy profit. To achieve this, I developed processes and procedures based on the SPECIAL formula that was simple to replicate across multiple locations.

Is your practice SPECIAL?

Before we go forward, let's take a quick look at what SPECIAL means to the overall health of your practice.

Scheduling

There is nothing that wastes more time and money than inefficient scheduling. In order to maximize the return on your investment, you'll need to make your business as profitable as possible, and scheduling is a big part of that equation.

In my own business, I prioritized my scheduling based on the different categories of patients.

The first category is the patient with no insurance and will pay out of pocket right away. There is no time wasted on collections or dealing with insurance forms and bureaucracy.

The second tier on my scheduling list is older patients. Many of these are free from the financial obligations of kids and a mortgage and, therefore, have the means to focus on their own health and well-being - while also being more flexible for appointments.

The third tier of patients has a type of dental insurance that's becoming increasingly hard to find - allowing the dentist to balance bill. That means if I have a fee of $100, the insurance company is going to pay $80 and the patient is responsible for that $20 balance.

The fourth tier of patients is covered under some type of government assistance, which basically means the government has a plan. The most familiar to practitioners is Medicaid, where they pay a flat fee for service and only certain services are covered.

The final tier is made up of those patients with insurance that does not permit balance billing. This means you have no control over what you're getting paid for procedures.

Prioritize you scheduling along these patient categories and you will see a difference on your balance sheet that will be very important when it comes to selling your practice.

Production

Focus on production to get your practice growing at the rate that makes it more attractive to buyers.

Create a production goal for your office each day. Whether you do it per hour, per appointment slot, or per day, it's crucially important to set benchmarks that lead to an overall monthly goal based on your overhead. If your scheduling was done well, then production should improve at a rate that buyers will notice.

Employees

When it comes to staff, I prefer to think of them as Team Members who have a deep connection to their jobs and your continued success.

The single most important factor that all successful practices have in common is training programs. A highly skilled team that is constantly improving skills will lead to better outcomes, happier patients, and more referrals. Again, this business growth will be important to potential buyers during the valuation process.

Collections

Collections, is part of every business - including dentistry. It's your business so it's your responsibility to understand that it's a successful billing process and procedure that keeps the doors open and the roof over your family's head. If you don't take collections seriously, you are undermining the stability of your investment and making it less attractive to buyers.

If your practice is collecting less than 97% of its billings, you need to improve. This can be done by engaging agencies such as Care Credit or Wells Fargo. These companies will provide the soft credit check so you can be confident that you are paid for the care and services you provide.

Internal controls

The best internal control is your signature. You sign the checks, and checks never leave the office without your signature. Once you lose control of that simple process, you're taking an unnecessary risk. When you are preparing your practice for sale, the last thing you are going to want is awkward revelations that reduce the value someone is willing to pay.

Associates

There will always be a ceiling to how many procedures you can perform in a single day. But increasing the number of procedures your practice can do shows on the balance sheet that potential buyers are looking at.

If you want to expand your business and make it attractive to purchasers, one of the best investments you can make is bringing on an associate.

Liability

When you are preparing to sell your practice, you need to know your exposure by maximizing your income vs liability.

Here are my basic guidelines. If you are not here now, then take the necessary steps to make it happen. The more attractive your numbers are, the better positioned you will be to maximize the return on your investment.

- Salaries should be between 25 and 28 percent.
- Supplies should be in the range of 5 percent
- Marketing should be between 2 and 4 percent.
- Dental lab should range between 6 and 10 percent.
- Rent and/or mortgage should be around 10 percent.
- Hardware and software should be around 5 percent.
- Insurance costs should be around 5 percent.

Overall, you want to position your practice so that overhead liabilities are below 70 percent. Of course, this is a guideline, and depending on your equipment and the type of practice you have, this can shift up and down significantly. But generally, 70 percent or less should be your goal when you are preparing for sale.

7 steps to getting the best value for your practice

Do you understand the environmental aspects of your office? There's the external environment, which is your socio-cultural, economic, regulatory, and ethical environments.

There's an operating environment, which deals with suppliers, patients, influence groups, allies, and income predators.

There's an internal environment, which is made up of organizational personnel, marketing, production, financial, and personal concerns.

And lastly, there are environmental goals to create the most successful clinical and financial practice for you and your team.

Understanding these four environments is critical. In most cases, I would strongly urge you start this process three to five years before you anticipate selling or merging your asset. After you've reviewed the different four stages outlined earlier, you have to go through a series of seven steps in order to get the best value for your practice.

Step 1. Develop your core values

My hope is at this stage in your dental practice, you've already determined your core values. These are basically made up of patient care objectives, quality of care, the work environment, your management style, team members and their responsibilities, professional growth for you and your team, a reward structure and a relationship with the community. Keep in mind the quality of care in your work environment is paramount. As potential owners look at your practice, they will take a significant look at the quality of care you've been providing and the work environment you've set up for your team members.

Step 2. Establish your practice mission

Core values are what you believe in, whereas a practice mission describes what you want your practice to accomplish. It's really a practice philosophy. Your mission statement is based on your attitudes and background, and should be written down to align with each core value.

The mission statement I created for my practice back in 1983 and still use today, is to be so good at what we do that our patients can't help but tell friends and family about our practice. Each of you will select not just your core values, but you should also have a mission statement that is clear so your team members know the common goal.

Step 3. Assess your environment

Apply the "SWOT" analysis to your practice.

Strengths
Weakness
Opportunities
Threats.

Write down your strengths, weaknesses, opportunities and threats, and in the next three to five years, tackle each of these so you have a clear analysis of your practice.

Step 4. Determine your strategies

Strategies should be well thought out and you should have a firm understanding of where you want to take your practice and team members.

Hopefully, most of your strategies are already well-developed. But if they need to be tweaked, revisit them. One of your strategies could include your plan for third party insurance plans. Are you accepting all insurances, and what particular plans are you rejecting versus accepting?

Revisit your credit and collection policies. Make sure your collections are above 98 percent, and if they are not, take a look at the weaknesses. Evaluate your fees and make sure they are up-to-date and competitive within your market area.

Take a hard look at your dental opportunities and infrastructure in your entire office situation. Keep in mind that if you're going to sell a home, curb appeal is critical to getting the best value – and is the quickest way to sell that home.

Get your facility in tiptop shape. Take a look at your hours of operation. Are you open evenings and Saturdays? Is your office convenient for new patients? Keep in mind as you prepare your practice for acquisition or sale, it's critical that your facility be open to and capable of, accepting new patients.

Evaluate yourself and your team's continuing education. Are you up to date on the latest care and treatment for TMD disorders? Sleep medicine? Botox dermal fills? Fixed and removable prostheses? Implant surgery and prostheses?

Having these skills as part of your package only increases the value of your practice to potential buyers and that's why I am a passionate advocate for continuous improvement through education and team skills development.

Step 5. Set goals and objectives

Aim to have your practice in the best shape possible before showing it off to prospective buyers. Is your practice actually profitable? What is your overhead? Are you able to get your overhead under 70 percent? Do you have a reasonable workload? Are you seeing a fair amount of patients in a variety of different clinical areas? You should be able to show prospective buyers that you're offering a wide variety of treatment to prove your practice is in the best position to receive the greatest return on investment possible. Are your patients happy and satisfied? Do you have appropriate quality assurance quality assessment?

Google searches and reviews indicating that your practice is not only well run, but also the marketing behind it is up to date and more than satisfactory, is also an important indicator. Is your practice involved in the community? Is the community even aware of your practice? The list can go on and on, but it is critical that there be some kind of tangible attachment between you and your community to provide the best value for your practice.

Step 6. Develop methods to increase your marketing

Look at your marketing and advertising. Do you have a system that is generating new patients and improving the bottom line of your practices? Develop methods to achieve your marketing goals. Your goal for a solo practice should be at least 40 to 50 new patients a month. If you need to expand the hours of operation and accept additional plans, do so.

Understanding that the acquisition and sale of your practice will in most cases be to an individual who will need to expand hours, to cover the initial investment means that you need to show there is room to grow and expand.

Step 7. Measure your metrics

You need to know exactly how many new patients you're receiving each month and where they're coming from. You also should know how many patients are leaving your practice and why. Also, create reports on the number of procedures that you're doing each month. These metrics are important information that buyers are going to be very interested in. The further back you have them, the better. This is why I say that it is so important to start preparing for your transition 3-5 years out.

Other critical information you need to have includes your net production and net collection.

The most crucial is knowing your EBITDA. This stands for Earnings Before Interest Taxes Depreciation. If you're thinking of selling to a dental service organization (DSO) or managed service organization(MSO), it's critical that you not only know what the EBITDA is, but also that you fully understand it because many times large groups that will be acquiring your practice will be looking for that calculation.

We all create treatment plans, but very few practices actually understand and evaluate how many of these plans are accepted and followed through. If your percentage of acceptance is low, you may want to take a look at how it's being explained and how you're marketing yourself in this care.

Some other considerations

- Do you need to hire or terminate team members who have been hanging on and not actually providing value to your practice? Is your practice set up to accommodate the new potential owner or will the new owner partner with you? Keep in mind that in most cases, the new owner will likely ask you to stay on for 6 to 24 months — or even longer to see the transition through. In most cases, you will get a much better return on your investment if you are willing to stay on.

- Take a look at your team members' compensation and make sure that it's up to date and competitive. Evaluate the benefits for your team members, which should include medical, dental, life disability, CPR, and continuing education. Take a look at your financial situation. Are you in a position to sell this practice and do you know what kind of money is necessary to put you in a position so that you can enjoy your retirement?

- Take a look at your fees and make sure that they are adequate, that they don't need to be lowered or increased. Make a keen evaluation of your credit policies, are your accounts receivable in line? The rule of 45 days simply states that you should have 45 days of accounts receivable. If your practice does $100,000 a month, or 1.2 million a year, 45 days of accounts receivable would be roughly $150,000. If your accounts receivable is significantly less than the 45-day rule, your credit and financial policies may be too stringent. If your accounts receivable is significantly higher than the rule of 45, then your business acumen or front desk may not be as good as you think.

- Lastly, you want to know about the cash flow. What is the profit? Has it been increasing, decreasing or staying static over the last few years? Most prospective buyers are going to want to look at a picture of three to five years past to see what the average success of your practice has been. That's why you should run your practice efficiently right from the start. But in reality, most people don't pay attention for about 12 to 24 months prior to deciding they're going to sell.

You have to fully understand what makes your dental practice profitable.

You have to understand how to manage an efficient and effective operation. You must also understand how you're managing your risk. These factors are critical for you to review and make sure you're comfortable so that you can achieve the best return on your investment.

But in the real world, we let things slip through the cracks day to day. Make an effort to understand not just the stages of your practice, but the steps to make it successful. What's the value of your practice and how is that value determined?

Value vs. price

Remember this: value does not equal price. Value is an estimate of financial worth of a practice, usually determined by formulas. Price, however, is determined by the how-much-the-seller-wants-to-sell and how-much-the-buyer-wants-to-buy rule.

Gross production is not what you want to sell your practice for. You may hope you can, but in reality, a savvy buyer will not want to purchase on gross production. A much better determinant to decide the value of your practice is based on net income, as shown on a tax return.

Be prepared to provide three to five years of tax returns – federal and state – to the prospective buyer. What a buyer is looking for is to purchase a dental practice based on its ability to make a profit. The seller, if they truly understand this, should make this their number one goal every day in preparation for the eventual sale.

Future profits are not written in stone, so individuals are generally looking at the value or price of the practice as it is today - not what it might be 10 years from now.

When I lecture and discuss these issues with various groups, I always recommend creating the greatest amount of profit for your practice. That will give you the best value when selling off your practice, an asset.

There are a variety of methods of valuing assets that you should understand. These include:

- The fair market value
- The replacement value
- The book value
- The economic depreciation

I won't go into great depth, but just understand that when we're talking about assets, those are the four basic methods of valuing an asset.

There are also four-asset classifications you need to understand. These are:

- **Tangible assets.** These include consumables such as furniture fixtures, leasehold improvements, and physical assets. Tangible assets are generally going to be a small part of the value of your practice.
- **Intangible assets**. These are usually made up of goodwill, restrictive covenant, ongoing concern, or value.
- **Financial assets.** This is the cash on hand security deposits and accounts receivable.
- **Real estate assets.** This is the land or the building at which the practice is on.

You should take a look at these four asset classifications and be able to determine the value or price for each of these assets in your practice.

Understanding your assets

Consider a reputable equipment dealer or expert to put a price or fair market value on your equipment and supplies. Another method that's quicker, is to consider for each doctor or hygienist, there's approximately $5,000 worth of supplies and equipment. So if there's a two-doctor practice and two hygienists, you probably have close to $20,000 in tangible assets.

Assets are generally depreciated in the intangible asset class of over 15 years. Goodwill will generally make up between 65 and 75 percent of the cost of a practice. But keep in mind your focus is the profitability of the practice.

Financial assets are generally accounts receivable. The zero to 30 days, I suggest that anywhere between 85 and 95 percent fee paid those accounts receivable between 30 and 60 days. I suggest getting 75 to 80 percent of that value accounts receivable 60 to 90 days will have a much lower value of usually 50 to 75 percent, and accounts receivable from 90 to 100 days approximately zero to 30 percent and any dollars owed over 120 days.

In most cases, there will be no value for those accounts receivable over 120 days unless there are extenuating circumstances. Your options when dealing with the financial assets, and in particular accounts receivable, are the buyer collects them or the seller collects them. If the office has a generally high collection rate of between 98 99 percent, I suggest paying the higher range on the accounts receivable.

If the office has a lower collection rate, less than 95 percent, I would suggest the lower percentage on the 30 to 90-day accounts receivable. Any accounts receivable 90 days and over should no longer be considered in the equation.

Lastly, make sure your lease is up to date so the potential buyer will not have any hang-ups with the existing owner or the lease agreement. I strongly emphasize that these leases should be at least five to seven years at length and should have acceptable terms. Do everything in your power to upgrade your lease terms to improve the sale and the return that you're going to get from your practice if the real estate is owned. I suggest a separate loan dealing with just the real estate based on an appraised value. In many cases, I would suggest two or three different appraisals and take the average of that to get a fair appraisal of the real estate.

If you are the dentist or the owner, there are a variety of methods of evaluating your practice. There's the **Summation of Asset Method** the **Profit Capitalization Method** the **Comparable Sales Method** and the **Cash Flow Feasibility Method (CFFM)**.

Although these names have a variety of different expertise behind them, in accounting, the **CFFM** is, in my opinion, the most appropriate method to improve the valuation of your practice.

The **CFFM** involves simply looking at your revenue, subtracting normal business expenses, taxes family budget expenses, and retirement plan contributions.

This will leave you the income available for debt service cash flow associated with the loan terms and interest rates. It should tell the buyer whether they can afford the purchase price or not. And if they can, will they be able to service the debt and still make an adequate living?

Using this method, you will see whether your asking price is accurate and fair. The way you price your practice based on this information will determine the speed at which you are able to sell your asset.

The calculation of the CFFM should be done three to five years before you are ready to sell. This will help you determine what is needed to help you get to the maximum value. Three to five years isn't a long time. But you can make a lot of corrections and undo a lot of bad mistakes, and increase the profitability of your practice significantly during that period.

Most of us will focus on the actual price, but keep in mind that the way the practice is sold, how the assets are handled, and how the taxes are actually addressed may sometimes have a bigger impact than the actual purchase price from the seller's perspective. The critical issue is to get as much of the purchase price to be goodwill as possible.

In summary, the seller's goal is to have as much of the purchase price go towards the long-term capital gain. Earlier, I discussed that in many cases, 65 to 75 percent of the actual purchase price will be attributed to goodwill from a buyer's perspective. Some of the money will go towards supplies and will be deducted in a 12-month period due to depreciation. Other money will go towards capital assets or long-term assets and deductions can still be made along with depreciation. But this is generally over a longer period of time of three to seven years.

The intangible assets, which in many cases are the biggest portion of the purchase price for the prospective buyer, are generally done over 15 years. So the buyers' goal is to have as much of the purchase price allocated towards supplies or tangible assets for a faster depreciation and higher cash flow. So you can see from the tax implications that the seller and the buyer have two different objectives. In general, keeping to the formula of 65 to 75 percent of the purchase price being goodwill is a relatively good compromise for both parties.

Another option to consider is managed service organizations and dental service organizations. Regardless of your personal feelings, these companies have the expertise and the financial backing that can make your transitions less stressful and much simpler.

However, understand that we're minnows swimming with sharks. The men and women who are part of managed service organizations have a financial background, and they acquire businesses for a living.

If you're not sure, you have to become very confident quickly that your business is in the best position to give you the highest value when dealing with managed service or dental service organizations.

The distinction, in my opinion, is managed service organizations are generally backed by equity groups or venture capitalists, whereas dental service organizations are generally practices that are owned and operated by dentists and generally have more than a couple of dental practices or an acquisition under their belt.

Keep in mind the difference is significant for managed service organizations as they generally have a shorter timeframe in their sites. They're trying to triple or quadruple their investment in three to seven years, whereas a dental service organization may have a much longer strategic plan.

Managed service organizations and dental service organizations could be an excellent strategy for you to consider if you want to continue to practice without the stress and strain of management and decision making. Of course, you have to be comfortable with the notion that you are essentially becoming an employee to increase your income over the next several years as you transition from full-time owner to part time associate, or eventually full time retirement. As with most things in our dental profession, there is nothing that is tried and true.

Final thought

I hope this book has provided a foundation to make the transition from owner to seller as simple and as stress-free as possible. My goal was to provide you with the best processes, procedures, and information to help you reach the highest return on your investment.

If you would like to consult on how to sell your practice, you can find out more at ascent-dental-solutions.com.

10 principles of success

As we wrap up, I'd like you to focus in on what I consider the 10 most important principles for success not only for you professionally, but personally as well.

1. Create a vision. If you want true success, you have to have a vision for your practice and for yourself personally.

2. Have a code of conduct. You have to have a code of conduct no matter how much money you make, or how successful your business is. If you don't have a code of conduct and you put your patients' wants and needs ahead of yours - your success will be short-lived, your team will suffer and you will suffer.

3. Strong communication. When you think your patient understands what you said and you think your team members understand what you said, they likely didn't. Relentless communication is paramount to success.

4. Have a financial plan. As I say to the students in my practice management class, you have to have some kind of financial goal. If you're not sure what that goal is, start by putting away 10 percent of your income. It doesn't really matter what you do with that 10 percent. But you should get in the habit of saving that amount of money so that at some point in your life you're working because you want to, not because you have to.

5. Continue to raise the bar. You're either accelerating and improving or declining. There's no such thing as being static in business or in life. In order to achieve true success, aim to raise the bar. You can do this with continuing education courses, additional training in communication, sales, and marketing.

6. Be the final decision maker. You have to understand that you're the final decision maker no matter what your strengths or weaknesses are. You have an obligation to yourself, your patient base, and to your team members to be that final decision maker. And if you make a mistake (and most of us do), you shouldn't worry unless you don't correct it.

The sooner you make that course correction, the better off you and your team will be.

7. Never be embarrassed to solicit help and support. I can tell you not a day goes by where someone teaches me something I didn't know. Or that someone tells me I was doing something incorrectly or not as well as I should be. As my children said to me growing up, "Dad, how come you need to take more courses. Shouldn't you know everything by now?" And 35 years later? I still don't know it all and nobody ever will.

We all need mentors in our life, and the sooner you can surround yourself with excellent mentors, the better off your professional and personal life will be.

8. Demand excellence. Demand excellence not just from yourself but the people around you. Once you accept mediocrity in your personal or professional life, it will grow like cancer. You will feel unsuccessful and you will become unsuccessful. There is nothing wrong with demanding excellence, but keep in mind you have to have the processes and procedures in place so that the people around you can establish excellence too.

9. Implement and use technology. Never before has it been so easy to gather information and data to improve your personal and professional life. It surrounds us. It is ubiquitous. It is in our face. Take advantage of the technology. If you don't, you're doing yourself and your team a disservice.

10. Encourage continuous positive action. It's so easy for us to demean our team members. It takes a bigger, smarter, and a stronger person to focus on the positives, take a look at those negatives, and put in proper processes and procedures so that we can reduce, or hopefully eliminate, the negativity.

www.ingramcontent.com/pod-product-compliance
Lightning Source LLC
Chambersburg PA
CBHW071205220526
45468CB00003B/1169